Renal Diet Cookbook for Beginners 2021

The Low Sodium, Low Phosphorus and Low Potassium Healthy Cookbook for the Newly Diagnosed to Stop Kidney Disease and Avoid Dialysis

Jasmine Wilkinson

Table of Contents

Renal Diet: Definition And Benefits

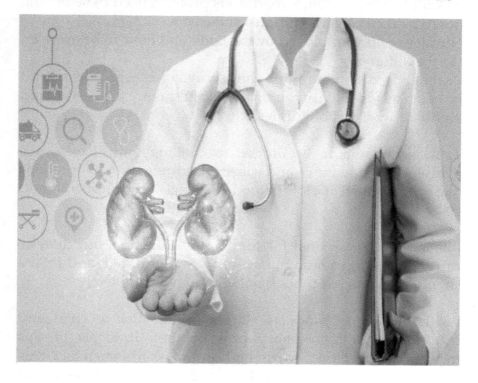

A renal diet is an eating plan designed to cause as little work or stress on the kidneys as possible, while still providing energy and the high nutrients the body needs.

A renal diet follows several fundamental guidelines.
The first is that it must be a balanced, healthy, and sustainable diet, rich in natural grains, vitamins, fibers, carbohydrates, omega 3 fats, and fluids. Proteins should be adequate, but not excessive.
Blood electrolyte levels must be monitored regularly, and the diet corrected. It is essential to follow specific advice from your doctor and dietitian.

Daily protein intake is essential to rebuild tissues but needs to be kept to a minimum. Superfluous proteins need to be broken down by the body into nitrates and carbs.

Nitrates are not employed by the body and have to be excreted via the kidneys.

Carbohydrates are an important source of energy and should be taken in adequate amounts. Whole grains are the best. Avoid highly refined carbohydrates.

Table salt ought to be limited to cooking only. Excess salt overworks the kidneys and causes fluid retention. Salty foods like processed meats, lots of foods, sausages, and snacks should be avoided.

Phosphorus is essential for the body to function, but dialysis can't remove it, so amounts need to be monitored, and intake should be restricted though not eliminated completely.

Foods, like dairy products, darker drinks such as colas and legumes, have high phosphorus content. If levels of this increase in the blood, foods high in potassium such as citrus fruits and dark, leafy green lettuce, carrots or apricots might have to be restricted.

Omega 3 fats are a significant part of any healthy diet. Fish is an excellent source. Omega fats are important for the body. Avoid trans-fats or hydrolyzed fats.

Fluids should be enough but might need to be limited in cases of fluid retention.

A healthy renal diet can help keep kidney function for longer.

The main differences between a renal diet and any nutritious diet plan are the limitations placed on protein and table salt ingestion. Restrictions on fluids and potassium might become necessary as signs and symptoms of accumulation become evident.

For people with kidney issues, they should eat less of these foods full of potassium, phosphorus and sodium. A blood sugar-lowering diet for people with diabetes can be a diet suitable for renal issues. Patients need to check labels since sodium is common in several foods.

All forms of renal diet have one thing in common, which is to improve your renal functions, bring some relief to your kidneys, as well as prevent kidneys disease at patients with numerous risk factors, altogether improving your overall health and wellbeing.

You don't need to shop many different types of groceries all at once as it is always better to use fresh produce, although frozen food also makes a good alternative when fresh fruit and vegetables are not available.

As far as the renal diet we are recommending in our guide, this form of kidney-friendly dietary regimen offer solution in form of low-sodium and low-potassium meals and groceries, which is why we are also offering simple and easy renal diet recipes in our guide.

Before we get to cooking and changing your lifestyle from the very core with the idea of improving your health, we want you to get familiar with renal diet basics and find out exactly what his diet is based on while you already know what is the very core solution found in renal diet - helping you improve your kidney's health by lowering sodium and potassium intake.

Phosphorus and How It Relates to Kidneys Disease

Phosphorus represents an essential mineral that serves the purpose of maintaining bone structure and taking care of bone cells development.

Phosphorus has more roles in our organism as an essential mineral, working on connective tissue repairment and enabling muscle movement. However, when concentrations of this mineral in your organism are too high as kidneys are unable to level phosphorus levels due to slow and damaged renal functions, redundant phosphorus becomes dangerous and may cause further health complications and aid in progression of your chronic kidney's disease.

Once phosphorus levels in your blood have surpassed recommended concentrations, the otherwise useful mineral becomes dangerous for your health as phosphorus then draws calcium from your bones, making the bones weak.

Common signs that appear as symptoms at kidney patients who have increased levels of phosphorus in their blood can appear in form of heart calcification, weak and easily breakable bones, muscle pain, as well as calcification of skin and joints, as well as blood vessel calcification.

With high levels of phosphorus that damaged kidneys are not able to eject from your blood, calcium builds up and can affect your lungs, eyes, heart and blood vessels, altogether bringing more damage to your renal functions that are already weakened.

That is why watching out for phosphorus levels beside monitoring levels of potassium and sodium is essential for your renal health and can be easily conducted through a suitable diet such as renal diet that originally prescribes low-sodium and low-potassium intake on a daily basis.

Just as it is the case with potassium and sodium, phosphorus is a mineral found in many different food groups, which means that intake of this essential mineral can be monitored through food consumption.

Phosphorus in Food: How to Lower Phosphorus Levels Through Renal Diet

As you may monitor your intake of potassium and sodium through restricting food groups that have high concentrations of these minerals, you can likewise make sure to introduce your body to healthy levels of phosphorus with an appropriate diet. The entire philosophy of lowering phosphorus levels that should be regulated by your kidneys is to lower the intake of foods that are rich in this mineral. We don't recommend to completely let go of phosphorus-rich food groups as your body still needs phosphorus regardless of the state of your kidneys. Consult with your doctor to find out more about phosphorus levels in your blood so you would know which food you may need to give up on.

Foods that normally have high concentrations of phosphorus are meat, cheese, dairy, seeds, soda, seeds and fast foods, so you may want to watch out for these food groups and make sure that your overall consumption of protein and dairy is restricted and limited just as it is the case with foods rich in sodium and potassium.

In case phosphorus levels found in your blood are higher than recommended according to your physician you are more likely to be advised to cut on meat and dairy portions, while meat also contains high concentrations of potassium.

Best way of monitoring quantities of phosphorus, potassium and sodium you are ingesting through your everyday diet is to limit the food groups that contain high concentrations of these minerals.

Beside from limiting foods that contain high levels of these minerals, you can also limit phosphorus introduced to your organism by cutting on portions that contain food that is high in phosphorus, sodium or potassium. Make sure to get familiar with which food groups contain highest concentrations of phosphorus, while eating fresh veggies and fruit may help you in case you have increased phosphorus in your blood.

Food that has more than 120 mg of phosphorus per serving is considered to be high-phosphorus food and should be introduced to your diet in limited amounts and in smaller portions, as well as it is the case with foods that are rich in potassium and sodium.

Phosphate: Consumption of phosphate becomes dangerous when kidney failure reaches 80% and goes to the 4th/5th stage of kidney failure. So, it is better to lower your phosphate intake by counting the calories and minerals.

Protein: Being on a renal diet, you should intake 0.75 kg protein per day. Good source of protein are eggs, milk, cheese, meat, nuts, and fish.

Potassium: After getting diagnosed, if your results show your potassium level is high in the blood, then you should restrict your potassium intake. Baked and fried potatoes are very high in potassium. Leafy greens, fruit juices are high in potassium. You can still enjoy vegetables that are low in potassium.

Sodium: Adding salt is very important in our food, but when you are suffering from kidney problems, you have to omit or minimize your salt intake. Too much sodium intake can trigger high blood pressure and fluid retention in the body. You need to find substitutes that help season your food. Herbs and spices that are extracted from plants are a good option. Using garlic, pepper, mustard can increase the taste of your food without adding any salt. Avoid artificial "salts" that are low in sodium because they are high in potassium, which is also dangerous for kidney health.

BREAKFAST

1. Oatmeal And Fruit Muffins

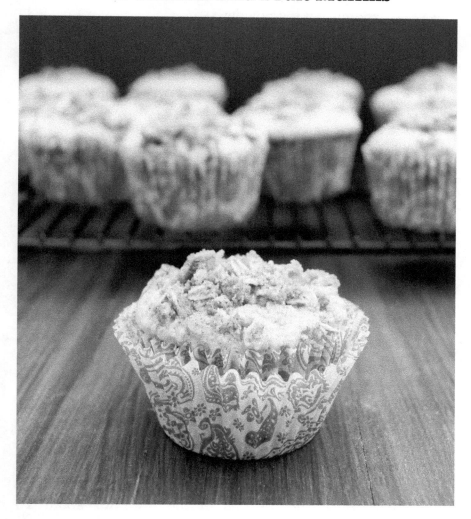

Preparation Time: 10 minutes
Cooking Time: 20 minutes
Servings: 4

Ingredients:

- 1 1/2 cup whole wheat bread flour or all-purpose
- 1 cup quick-cooking oatmeal
- 3/4 cups brown sugar whole or dark
- 2 teaspoons baking powder
- 1/2 teaspoon salt
- 1 cup sour cream 5% or 14%
- 2 teaspoons baking soda
- 1/2 cup canola oil
- 2 eggs
- 1 tablespoon vanilla extract
- 2 cups fresh or frozen fruit (blueberries, cherries, peaches, blackberries, strawberries, berries, etc.)

Directions:

1. Preheat the oven to 350 ¬∞ F. In a bowl, combine flour, oats, baking powder, and salt with a fork. Cut the fruit into 1 to 1.5 cm pieces if they are larger.
2. Meanwhile, mix the baking soda with the sour cream in a measuring cup of 2 cups. Allow swelling.
3. With an electric mixer, mix oil with eggs and vanilla. Add the brown sugar and mix well. Add swollen sour cream and mix gently.
4. Gradually add dry ingredients to moist ingredients. Mix gently between each addition. Add the fruits and mix with a spoon.
5. Divide the dough into muffin pans covered with paper boxes. Bake the muffins in the oven for about 20 minutes.

Nutrition:

- Calories: 127.2 kcal
- Total Fat: 5.3 g
- Saturated Fat: 0.2 g
- Cholesterol: 18.2 mg
- Sodium: 147.2 mg
- Total Carbs: 17.3 g
- Fiber: 2.1 g
- Sugar: 4.9 g
- Protein: 3.1 g

2. Breakfast With Avena Copos

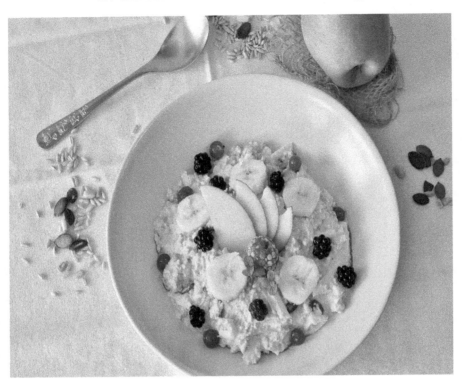

Preparation Time: 10 minutes
Cooking Time: 15 minutes
Servings: 4

Ingredients:

- 250 ml of milk (can be from a cow, soy, oatmeal, rice)
- 3 heaped tablespoons of oat flakes (I buy them at Mercadona)
- 1 tablespoon honey, sugar or cinnamon
- Half grated apple
- 1 handful of raisins
- Half banana cut
- 1 handful of walnuts, date chips, figs (any dried fruit)

Directions:

1. Put the milk in a saucepan with the oatmeal and simmer.
2. When it starts to boil, leave about 5 minutes (stirring so that it does not stick to you), finished those 5 minutes, let stand a few minutes with the fire off (it will be more fluffy).
3. Put in a bowl and add the sweetener that you want along with the apple, banana, and nuts.
4. you can take it both hot and cold.
5. NOTES:
6. You can take them if you want only with milk. Let's see that the important thing is to put the oatmeal flakes, and if we put more rich things, it is already a DELICIOUS AND HEALTHY BREAKFAST!

Nutrition:

- Calories: 338 kcal
- Total Fat: 6.8 g
- Saturated Fat: 1.3 g
- Cholesterol: 0 mg
- Sodium: 0.012 mg
- Total Carbs: 61 g
- Fiber: 0 g
- Sugar: 1 g
- Protein: 13 g

3. Banana Breakfast Pancakes

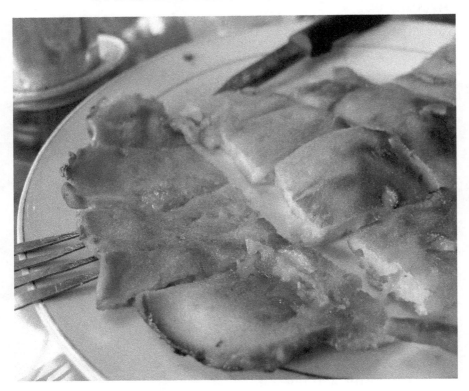

Preparation Time: 5 minutes
Cooking Time: 10 minutes
Servings: 3

Ingredients:

- ½ cup (63g.) Of wheat flour.
- ½ cup (80g.) Of flaked oatmeal.
- 2 small bananas (160g.) Mashed.
- 2 eggs (100g.).
- 1 cup (240g.) Ideal, 0% Fat, Evaporated Milk.
- 2 tablespoons (30g.) Brown sugar.
- 1 tablespoon (6g.) Of cinnamon.
- 1 teaspoon (5g.) Of butter.

Directions:

1. In a bowl, combine all ingredients, except butter.
2. In a pan over medium heat, place the butter and wait for it to melt.
3. Pour ¬° cup of the mixture over the pan and cook until it begins to bubble.
4. Turn the pancake and cook for 1 minute or until it browns on the other side.
5. Serve and enjoy.

Nutrition:

- Calories: 327.7 kcal
- Total Fat: 3.6 g
- Saturated Fat: 0.7 g
- Cholesterol: 0 mg
- Sodium: 2.2 mg
- Total Carbs: 58.5 g
- Fiber: 8.1 g
- Sugar: 0 g
- Protein: 15.3 g

4. Orange And Red Blueberry Cookies

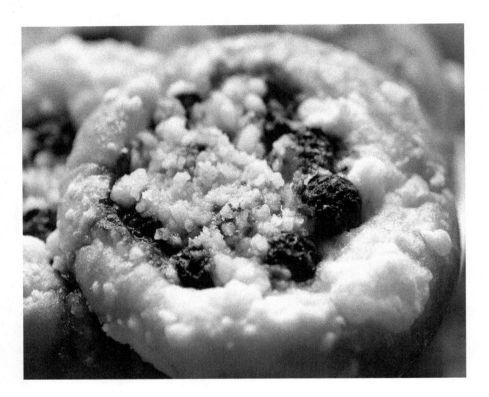

Preparation Time: 15 minutes
Cooking Time: 6 hours
Servings: 3

Ingredients:

- 4 T (360g) of oatmeal in fine flakes
- 2 T (250g without bone) dates
- 1 cheaped the vanilla powder
- 1 T (120g) dried cranberries
- 2 organic oranges (its juice and peel)
- sweet orange essence salt - optional
- 2 C mild oil (sunflower or almond) - optional

Directions:

1. Wash the oranges and grate them. Make the juice and reserve.
2. Crush the dates.
3. Put in the robot: oat flakes, dates, orange zest, vanilla, and a pinch of salt. Crush until it begins to stick, and dates have been chopped small.
4. Add the juice of the oranges and crush again to incorporate. (200ml at most, if you get a little less, nothing happens)
5. Now add the blueberries and mash - just a little, just enough for some to chop and others not.
6. Remove the robot and put it in a bowl.
7. Add the oil, although this is optional, if you do not have or do not want to put and the dough is sufficiently moistened so that you can form the cookies, you can skip it.
8. Make the cookies and put on the dehydrator tray. They do not need to be on teflex sheet or baking paper. I leave them as-is for the air to circulate better and be done before. Set the first hour at 52 degrees and the following at 42. They will be done in about 6 hours or so; after 4 hours, you can turn them around.

Nutrition:

- Calories: 58 kcal
- Total Fat: 2.3 g
- Saturated Fat: 0 g
- Cholesterol: 4 mg
- Sodium: 47 mg
- Total Carbs: 8.7 g
- Fiber: 0 g
- Sugar: 0 g
- Protein: 0.7 g

5. Tuna Spinach Sandwich

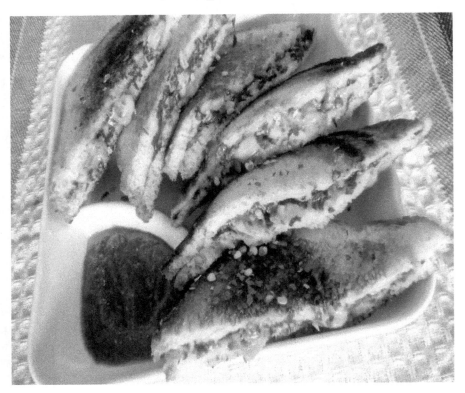

Preparation Time: 7 minutes
Cooking Time: 0 minute
Servings: 4

Ingredients:

The quantity of ingredients is to your liking and preference.

- Integral bread
- fresh and well-washed spinach
- tuna in well-drained water
- a ripe but firm avocado
- salt and pepper

Directions:

1. The spinach already washed and dried the short in thin strips, the finest you can.
2. What I do to achieve these strips is, I arrange several spinach leaves on top of each other, I make a small roll, and with a very sharp knife, I am cutting and thus they are excellent.
3. Avocado cut it into tiny cubes.
4. The bread is browned in a Teflon pan, on one side only.
5. Mix spinach with tuna and avocado.
6. Season the mixture with salt and pepper.
7. You put the stuffing in the bread and go.
8. Enjoy this delight.

Nutrition:

- Calories: 228 kcal
- Total Fat: 4.5 g
- Saturated Fat: 1.6 g
- Cholesterol: 24.7 mg
- Sodium: 779.4 mg
- Total Carbs: 26.8 g
- Fiber: 5.5 g
- Sugar: 3.3 g
- Protein: 24 g

6. Congee With Century Eggs

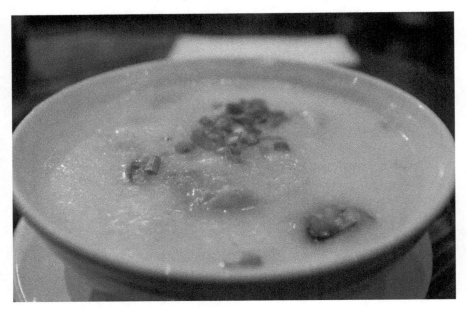

Preparation Time: 20 minutes
Cooking Time: 6 hours and 15 minutes
Servings: 6

Ingredients:

- 6 cups of water
- ½ cup red quinoa
- 2 garlic cloves, grated
- 2 large leeks, minced
- 1 tablespoon coconut oil
- 1 tablespoon brown rice, rinsed, drained
- ½ tablespoon dark soy sauce
- ¼ tablespoon low-sodium soy sauce
- Dash of garlic flakes
- ¼ tablespoon low-sodium teriyaki sauce
- ½ teaspoon ginger, grated
- ⅛ teaspoon white pepper
- ¼ pound ground lean beef
- Pinch of sea salt
- 2 large century eggs, boiled, quartered
- Dash of red pepper flakes

Directions:

1. Pour oil into non-stick skillet set over medium heat. Sauté leeks and garlic until limp and aromatic
2. add in beef. Stir-fry until meat browns
3. pour into slow cooker set at medium heat.
4. Except for garnishes, pour in remaining ingredients
5. stir. Put lid on. Cook for 6 hours. Turn off heat. Taste
6. adjust seasoning if needed.
7. Ladle congee into individual bowls. Garnish with leeks and century eggs. Sprinkle in garlic flakes and red pepper flakes. Cool slightly before serving.

Nutrition:

- Calories: 256 kcal
- Total Fat: 5 g
- Saturated Fat: 0 g
- Cholesterol: 0 mg
- Sodium: 0 mg
- Total Carbs: 39 g
- Fiber: 0 g
- Sugar: 0 g
- Protein: 10 g

7. Breakfast Cheesecake

Preparation Time: 10 minutes
Cooking Time: 20 minutes
Servings: 16

Ingredients:

- 4 eggs
- 7 cups Greek yogurt
- 7 cups cottage cheese
- 2 tablespoons honey, add more if needed
- 2 teaspoons vanilla
- ½ teaspoon olive oil
- ½ onion, chopped
- ½ cup uncured sausage
- Pinch of salt
- Pinch of pepper

Directions:

1. In a blender, combine eggs, cream cheese, cottage cheese, honey, and vanilla. Process until all ingredients are well combined.
2. Meanwhile, heat the olive oil in a pan. Sauté onion and uncured sausage. Season with salt and pepper. Cook for 4 minutes. Transfer the mixture into a baking dish.
3. Place inside the oven and bake for 10 minutes. Allow to cool at room temperature. Refrigerate for 1 hour before serving

Nutrition:

- Calories: 136.2 kcal
- Total Fat: 8 g
- Saturated Fat: 4.6 g
- Cholesterol: 85.1 mg
- Sodium: 319.3 mg
- Total Carbs: 6.3 g
- Fiber: 0 g
- Sugar: 0.1 g
- Protein: 11.3 g

SMOOTHIES

8. Winter Berry Smoothie

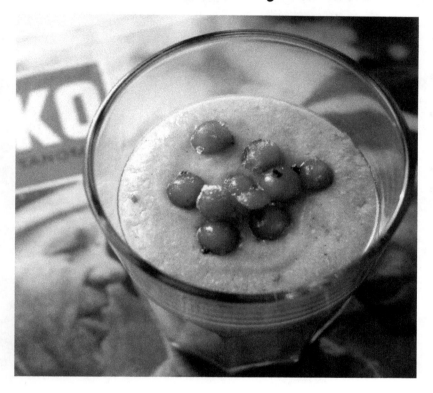

Preparation Time: 5 minutes
Cooking Time: 0 minute
Servings: 2

Ingredients:

- 1/4 cup blackberries
- 1/4 cup cherries, pitted
- 1/4 cup cranberries
- 2 cups water

Direction:

1. Blend until smooth in a blender or smoothie maker.
2. Serve right away.

Nutrition:

- Calories: 21 kcal
- Total Fat: 0 g
- Saturated Fat: 0 g
- Cholesterol: 0 mg
- Sodium: 1 mg
- Total Carbs: 5 g
- Fiber: 0 g
- Sugar: 0 g
- Protein: 2 g

9. Carrot Smoothie

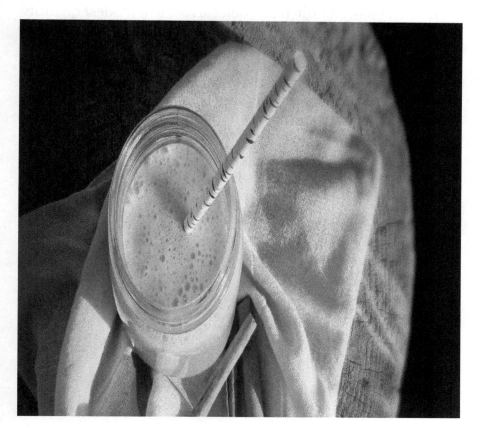

Preparation Time: 5 minutes
Cooking Time: 0 minute
Servings: 1

Ingredients

- 1 cup cut carrots
- ½ teaspoon finely destroyed orange strip
- 1 cup squeezed orange
- 1½ cups ice 3D shapes
- Orange strip twists (discretionary)

Directions:

1. In a secured little pan, cook carrots in a modest quantity of bubbling water around 15 minutes or until delicate. Channel well. Cool.
2. Spot depleted carrots in a blender. Include finely destroyed orange strip and squeezed orange.
3. Cover and mix until smooth.
4. Include ice blocks; cover and mix until smooth.
5. Fill glasses. Whenever wanted, decorate with orange strip twists.

Nutrition:

- Calories: 97 kcal
- Total Fat: 0.6 g
- Saturated Fat: 0.1 g
- Cholesterol: 0 mg
- Sodium: 28 mg
- Total Carbs: 22.4 g
- Fiber: 1.4 g
- Sugar: 17.3 g
- Protein: 0 g

10.   Strawberry Papaya Smoothie

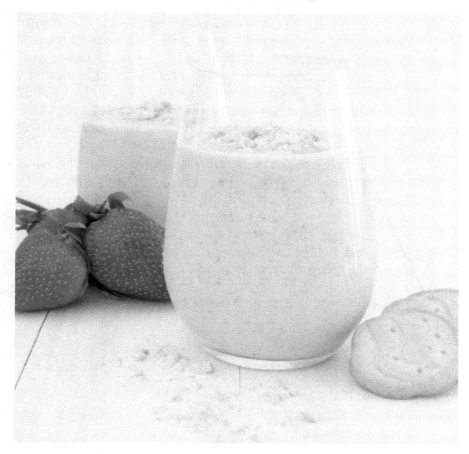

Preparation Time: 10 minutes
Cooking Time: 0 minute
Servings: 1

Ingredients:

- ½ cup of strawberries
- 2 cup of sliced papaya
- 2 cup of coconut kefir
- 2 scoop of vanilla bone broth protein powder
- ½ cup of ice water

Directions:

1. Did you realize that papaya is incredible for digestion? The tropical organic product is stacked with compounds and cell reinforcements that help the body detox and decrease irritation. It's likewise a too delectable element for smoothies. In case you're hoping to switch up your typical formula, it's a great opportunity to attempt this Strawberry Papaya Smoothie. You will need to add all the above ingredients to blender & blend on high.
2. This beverage is without dairy and utilizations coconut kefir for the help of a probiotic. At the point when blended in with vanilla protein powder and crisp strawberries, you have a simple, in a hurried breakfast or post-exercise supper to fuel your body.
3. Add every one of the ingredients to the blender, and mix until the Strawberry Papaya Smoothie is pleasantly joined. I love including a crisp sprig of mint to supplement this new and fruity smoothie.

Nutrition:

- Calories: 196.9 kcal
- Total Fat: 1.5 g
- Saturated Fat: 0.8 g
- Cholesterol: 43.6 mg
- Sodium: 152 mg
- Total Carbs: 28 g
- Fiber: 2.5 g
- Sugar: 14.5 g
- Protein: 19.6 g

11.   Gut Cleansing Smoothie

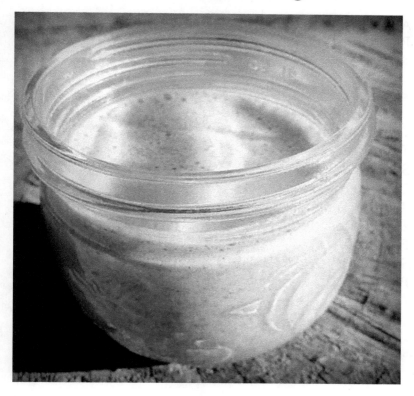

Preparation Time: 10 minutes
Cooking Time: 0 minute
Servings: 1

Ingredients:

- 1 ½ tablespoons coconut oil, unrefined
- ½ cup plain full-fat yogurt
- 1 tablespoon chia seeds
- 1 serving aloe vera leaves
- ½ cup frozen blueberries, unsweetened
- 1 tablespoon hemp hearts
- 1 cup of water
- 1 scoop Pinnaclife prebiotic fiber

Directions:

1. Add listed ingredients to a blender
2. Blend until you have a smooth and creamy texture
3. Serve chilled and enjoy!

Nutrition:

- Calories: 409 kcal
- Total Fat: 33 g
- Saturated Fat: 0 g
- Cholesterol: 0 mg
- Sodium: 0 mg
- Total Carbs: 8 g
- Fiber: 0 g
- Sugar: 0 g
- Protein: 12 g

12.   Cabbage And Chia Glass

Preparation Time: 10 minutes
Cooking Time: 0 minute
Servings: 2

Ingredients:

- 1/3 cup cabbage
- 1 cup cold unsweetened almond milk
- 1 tablespoon chia seeds
- ½ cup cherries
- ½ cup lettuce

Directions:

1. Add coconut milk to your blender
2. Cut cabbage and add to your blender
3. Place chia seeds in a coffee grinder and chop to powder, brush the powder into a blender
4. Pit the cherries and add them to the blender
5. Wash and dry the lettuce and chop
6. Add to the mix
7. Cover and blend on low followed by medium
8. Taste the texture and serve chilled!

Nutrition:

- Calories: 409 kcal
- Total Fat: 33 g
- Saturated Fat: 0 g
- Cholesterol: 0 mg
- Sodium: 0 mg
- Total Carbs: 8 g
- Fiber: 0 g
- Sugar: 0 g
- Protein: 12 g

13.   Almonds And Zucchini Smoothie

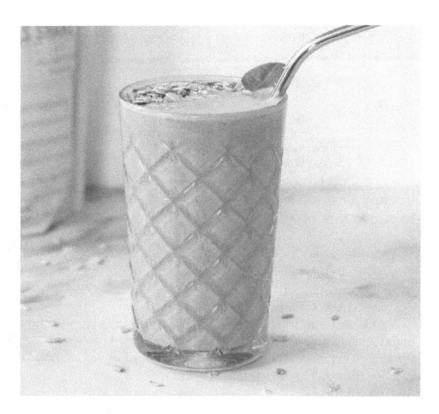

Preparation Time: 5 minutes
Cooking Time: 0 minute
Servings: 2

Ingredients:

- 1 cup zucchini, cooked and mashed - unsalted
- 1 1/2 cups almond milk
- 1 Tbsp almond butter (plain, unsalted)
- 1 tsp pure almond extract
- 2 Tbsp ground almonds or Macadamia almonds
- 1/2 cup water
- 1 cup Ice cubes crushed (optional, for serving)

Directions:

1. Dump all Ingredients from the list above in your fast-speed blender; blend for 45 - 60 seconds or to taste.
2. Serve with crushed ice.

Nutrition:

- Calories: 322 kcal
- Total Fat: 30 g
- Saturated Fat: 0 g
- Cholesterol: 0 mg
- Sodium: 0 mg
- Total Carbs: 6 g
- Fiber: 3.5 g
- Sugar: 0 g
- Protein: 6 g

,

14.   Baby Spinach And Dill Smoothie

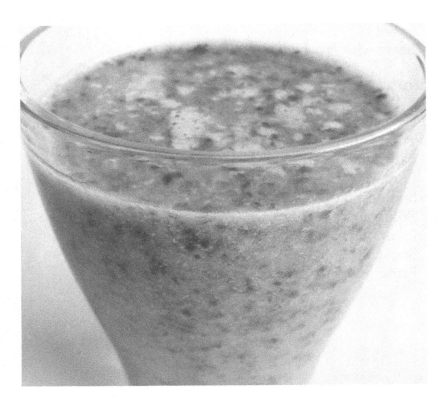

Preparation Time: 5 minutes
Cooking Time: 0 minute
Servings: 2

Ingredients:

- 1 cup of fresh baby spinach leaves
- 2 Tbsp of fresh dill, chopped
- 1 1/2 cup of water
- 1/2 avocado, chopped into cubes
- 1 Tbsp chia seeds (optional)
- 2 Tbsp of natural sweetener Stevia or Erythritol (optional)

Directions:

1. Place all Ingredients into fast-speed blender. Beat until smooth and all Ingredients united well.
2. Serve and enjoy!

Nutrition:

- Calories: 136 kcal
- Total Fat: 10 g
- Saturated Fat: 0 g
- Cholesterol: 0 mg
- Sodium: 0 mg
- Total Carbs: 8 g
- Fiber: 9 g
- Sugar: 0 g
- Protein: 7 g

SNACKS AND SIDES

15. Eggplant And Chickpea Bites

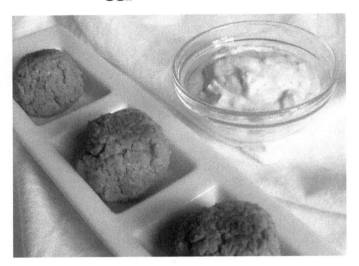

Preparation Time: 20 minutes
Cooking Time: 1 hour
Servings: 4

Ingredients:

- 3 large aubergines cut in half
- (make a few cuts in the flesh with a knife) Spray
- oil
- 2 large cloves garlic, peeled and deglazed
- 2 tbsp. coriander powder
- 2 tbsp. cumin seeds
- 400 g canned chickpeas, rinsed and drained
- 2 Tbsp. chickpea flour
- Zest and juice of 1/2 lemon
- 1/2 lemon quartered for serving
- 3 tbsp. tablespoon of polenta

Directions:

1. Heat the oven to 200¬ſC (180¬ſC rotating heat, gas level 6). Spray the eggplant halves generously with oil and place them on the meat side up on a baking sheet. Sprinkle with coriander and cumin seeds, and then place the cloves of garlic on the plate. Season and roast for 40 minutes until the flesh of eggplant is completely tender. Reserve and let cool a little.
2. Scrape the flesh of the eggplant in a bowl with a spatula and throw the skins in the compost. Thoroughly scrape and make sure to incorporate spices and crushed roasted garlic. Add chickpeas, chickpea flour, zest, and lemon juice. Crush roughly and mix well, check to season. Do not worry if the mixture seems a bit soft - it will firm up in the fridge.
3. Form about twenty pellets and place them on a baking sheet covered with parchment paper. Let stand in the fridge for at least 30 minutes.
4. Preheat oven to 180¬ſC (rotating heat 160¬ſC, gas level 4). Remove the meatballs from the fridge and coat them by rolling them in the polenta. Place them back on the baking sheet and spray a little oil on each. Roast for 20 minutes until golden and crisp. Serve with lemon wedges. You can also serve these dumplings with a spicy yogurt dip with harissa, this delicious but spicy mashed paste of hot peppers and spices from the Maghreb.

Nutrition:

- Calories: 178 kcal
- Total Fat: 39.4 g
- Saturated Fat: 0 g
- Cholesterol: 0 mg
- Sodium: 0 mg
- Total Carbs: 113 g
- Fiber: 0 g
- Sugar: 0 g
- Protein: 25.7 g

16.   Popcorn With Sugar And Spice

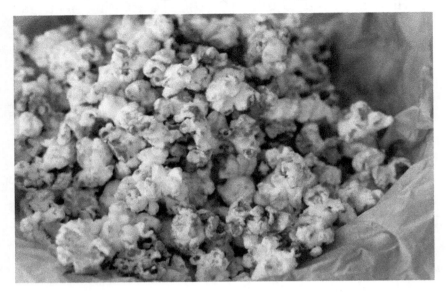

Preparation Time: 5 minutes
Cooking Time: 10 minutes
Servings: 3

Ingredients:

- 8 cups hot popcorn
- 2 tablespoons unsalted butter
- 2 tablespoons sugar
- 1/2 teaspoon cinnamon
- 1/4 teaspoon nutmeg

Directions:

1. Popping the corn; put aside.
2. Heat the butter, sugar, cinnamon, and nutmeg in the microwave or saucepan over a range fire until the butter is melted and the sugar dissolved.
3. Be careful not to burn the butter.
4. Sprinkle the corn with the spicy butter, mix well.
5. Serve immediately for optimal flavor.

Nutrition:

- Calories: 120 kcal
- Total Fat: 7 g
- Saturated Fat: 0 g
- Cholesterol: 16 mg
- Sodium: 2 mg
- Total Carbs: 12 g
- Fiber: 2.5 g
- Sugar: 0 g
- Protein: 2 g

17.   Baba Ghanouj

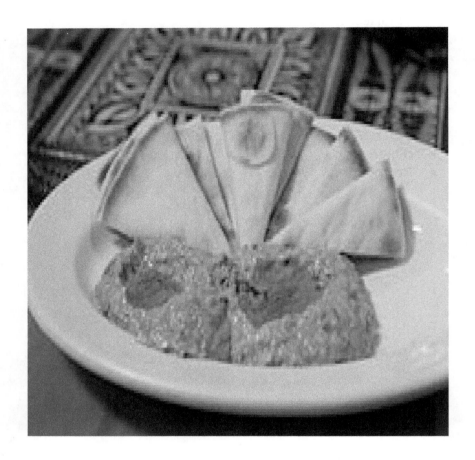

Preparation Time: 10 minutes
Cooking Time: 30 minutes
Servings: 4

Ingredients:

- 1 large aubergine, cut in half lengthwise
- 1 head of garlic, unpeeled
- 30 ml (2 tablespoons) of olive oil
- Lemon juice to taste

Directions:

1. Put the grill at the center of the oven. Preheat the oven to 350 F. Line a baking sheet with parchment paper.
2. Place the eggplant on the plate, skin side up. Roast until the meat is very tender and detaches easily from the skin, about 1 hour depending on the size of the eggplant. Let cool.
3. Meanwhile, cut the tip of the garlic cloves. Place the garlic cloves in a square
4. of aluminum foil. Fold the edges of the sheet and fold together to form a tightly wrapped foil. Roast with the eggplant until tender, about 20 minutes. Let cool. Purée the pods with a garlic press.
5. With a spoon, scoop out the flesh of the eggplant and place it in the bowl of a food processor. Add the garlic puree, the oil, and the lemon juice. Stir until purée is smooth and pepper.
6. Serve with mini pita bread.

Nutrition:

- Calories: 110 kcal
- Total Fat: 0 g
- Saturated Fat: 2.5 g
- Cholesterol: 10 mg
- Sodium: 180 mg
- Total Carbs: 1 g
- Fiber: 0 g
- Sugar: 0 g
- Protein: 1 g

,

18.   Baked Pita Chips

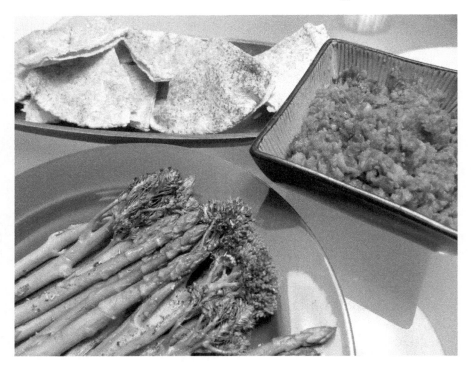

Preparation Time: 5 minutes
Cooking Time: 15 minutes
Servings: 6

Ingredients:

- 3 pita loaves (6 inches)
- 3 tablespoons olive oil
- Chili powder

Directions:

1. Separate each bread in half with scissors, to obtain 6 round pieces. Cut each piece into eight points.
2. Brush each with olive oil and sprinkle with chili powder. Bake at 350 degrees F for about 15 minutes until crisp.

Nutrition:

- Calories: 120 kcal
- Total Fat: 2.5 g
- Saturated Fat: 0 g
- Cholesterol: 0 mg
- Sodium: 70 mg
- Total Carbs: 22 g
- Fiber: 1 g
- Sugar: 0 g
- Protein: 3 g

19.   Almond And Pecan Caramel Popcorn

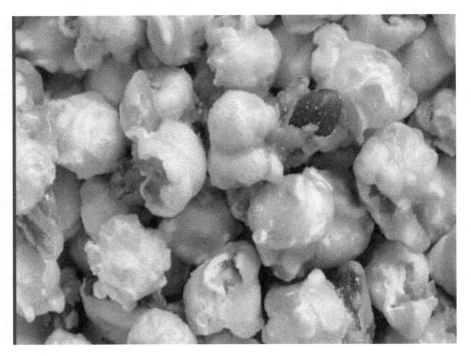

Preparation Time: 5 minutes
Cooking Time: 10 minutes
Servings: 10

Ingredients:

- 2 cups of unblanched almonds
- 8 oz of pecan halves
- 20 cups of popped popcorn
- 8 oz of granulated sugar
- 1 tsp. of sodium bicarbonate
- Pinch of cream of tartar
- 8 oz of unsalted butter
- 4 oz of corn syrup

Directions:

1. Using a large roasting pan, layer the popcorn evenly with the almonds and pecans.
2. Using a saucepan, stir together the sugar, butter, cream of tartar, and corn syrup. Cook the contents of the pan using a rolling bubble for five min. without stirring.
3. Combine with the soda after removing from the stove.
4. Drizzle over the nuts and popcorn. Stirring it to coat the popcorn and nuts well.
5. Bake at 200 for one hour, stirring it every ten minutes. Let cool, still stirring every ten minutes. Store for up to one week.

Nutrition:

- Calories: 604 kcal
- Total Fat: 6 g
- Saturated Fat: 0 g
- Cholesterol: 0 mg
- Sodium: 149 mg
- Total Carbs: 51 g
- Fiber: 4 g
- Sugar: 0 g
- Protein: 8 g

20.   Peanut Butter Balls

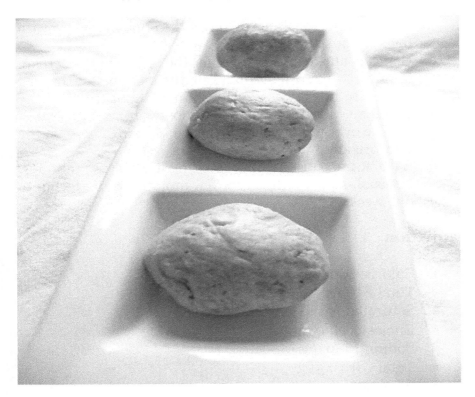

Preparation Time: 1 hour
Cooking Time: 0 minutes
 Servings: 12

Ingredients:

- 24 Tbsp. of graham cracker crumbs
- 8 oz cream cheese (low in fat)
- .5 cup of unsalted and unsweetened peanut butter
- .25 cup of mini chocolate chips
- 1 tsp. of vanilla
- .5 cup of shredded coconut

Directions:

1. With the exception of the coconut, combine all of the listed ingredients. Ensure they are completely combined.
2. Form into one-inch balls. Roll in the coconut.
3. Refrigerate for a minimum of one hour, or until they are firm. Store refrigerated seven days for put in freezer to enjoy later.

Nutrition:

- Calories: 150 kcal
- Total Fat: 0 g
- Saturated Fat: 0 g
- Cholesterol: 0 mg
- Sodium: 120 mg
- Total Carbs: 13 g
- Fiber: 0 g
- Sugar: 0 g
- Protein: 4 g

SOUPS AND STEWS

21. Spaghetti Squash & Yellow Bell-Pepper Soup

Preparation time: 10 minutes
Cooking time: 45 minutes
Servings: 4

Ingredients:

- 2 diced yellow bell peppers
- 2 chopped large garlic cloves
- 1 peeled and cubed spaghetti squash
- 1 quartered and sliced onion
- 1 tbsp. dried thyme
- 1 tbsp. coconut oil
- 1 tsp. curry powder
- 4 cups water

Direction:

1. Heat the oil in a large pan over medium-high heat before sweating the onions and garlic for 3-4 minutes.
2. Sprinkle over the curry powder.
3. Add the stock and bring to a boil over a high heat before adding the squash, pepper and thyme.
4. Turn down the heat, cover and allow to simmer for 25-30 minutes.
5. Continue to simmer until squash is soft if needed.
6. Allow to cool before blitzing in a blender/food processor until smooth.
7. Serve!

Nutrition:

- Calories: 103 kcal
- Total Fat: 4 g
- Saturated Fat: 0 g
- Cholesterol: 0 mg
- Sodium: 32 mg
- Total Carbs: 17 g
- Fiber: 0 g
- Sugar: 0 g
- Protein: 2 g

22.   Red Pepper & Brie Soup

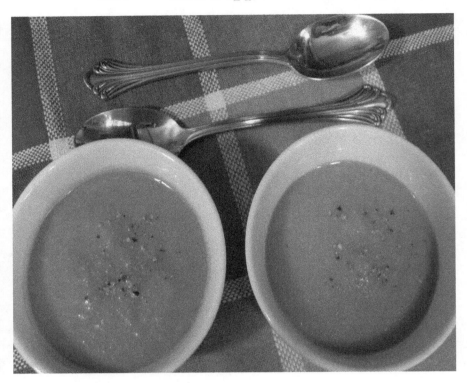

Preparation time: 10 minutes
Cooking time: 35 minutes
Servings: 4

Ingredients:

- 1 tsp. paprika
- 1 tsp. cumin
- 1 chopped red onion
- 2 chopped garlic cloves
- ¬⁰ cup crumbled brie
- 2 tbsps. extra virgin olive oil
- 4 chopped red bell peppers
- 4 cups water

Direction:

1. Heat the oil in a pot over medium heat.
2. Sweat the onions and peppers for 5 minutes.
3. Add the garlic cloves, cumin and paprika and sauté for 3-4 minutes.
4. Add the water and allow to boil before turning the heat down to simmer for 30 minutes.
5. Remove from the heat and allow to cool slightly.
6. Put the mixture in a food processor and blend until smooth.
7. Pour into serving bowls and add the crumbled brie to the top with a little black pepper.
8. Enjoy!

Nutrition:

- Calories: 152 kcal
- Total Fat: 11 g
- Saturated Fat: 0 g
- Cholesterol: 0 mg
- Sodium: 66 mg
- Total Carbs: 8 g
- Fiber: 0 g
- Sugar: 0 g
- Protein: 3 g

,

23. Turkey & Lemon-Grass Soup

Preparation time: 5 minutes
Cooking time: 40 minutes
Servings: 4

Ingredients:

- 1 fresh lime
- ¼ cup fresh basil leaves
- 1 tbsp. cilantro
- 1 cup canned and drained water chestnuts
- 1 tbsp. coconut oil
- 1 thumb-size minced ginger piece
- 2 chopped scallions
- 1 finely chopped green chili
- 4oz. skinless and sliced turkey breasts
- 1 minced garlic clove, minced
- ½ finely sliced stick lemon-grass
- 1 chopped white onion, chopped
- 4 cups water

Direction:

1. Crush the lemon-grass, cilantro, chili, 1 tbsp oil and basil leaves in a blender or pestle and mortar to form a paste.
2. Heat a large pan/wok with 1 tbsp olive oil on high heat.
3. Sauté the onions, garlic and ginger until soft.
4. Add the turkey and brown each side for 4-5 minutes.
5. Add the broth and stir.
6. Now add the paste and stir.
7. Next add the water chestnuts, turn down the heat slightly and allow to simmer for 25-30 minutes or until turkey is thoroughly cooked through.
8. Serve hot with the green onion sprinkled over the top.

Nutrition:

- Calories: 123 kcal
- Total Fat: 3 g

- Saturated Fat: 0 g
- Cholesterol: 0 mg
- Sodium: 501 mg
- Total Carbs: 12 g
- Fiber: 0 g
- Sugar: 0 g
- Protein: 10 g

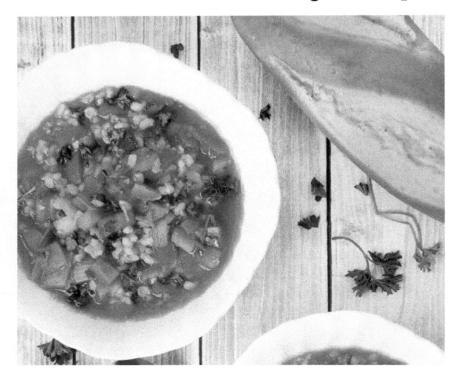

Preparation time: 5 minutes
Cooking time: 30 minutes
Servings: 4

Ingredients:

- 1 tbsp. oregano
- 2 minced garlic cloves
- 1 tsp. black pepper
- 1 diced zucchini
- 1 cup diced eggplant
- 4 cups water
- 1 diced red pepper
- 1 tbsp. extra-virgin olive oil
- 1 diced red onion

Direction:

1. Soak the vegetables in warm water prior to use.
2. In a large pot, add the oil, chopped onion and minced garlic.
3. Sweat for 5 minutes on low heat.
4. Add the other vegetables to the onions and cook for 7-8 minutes.
5. Add the stock to the pan and bring to a boil on high heat.
6. Stir in the herbs, reduce the heat, and simmer for a further 20 minutes or until thoroughly cooked through.
7. Season with pepper to serve.

Nutrition:

- Calories: 152 kcal
- Total Fat: 3 g
- Saturated Fat: 0 g
- Cholesterol: 0 mg
- Sodium: 3 mg
- Total Carbs: 6 g
- Fiber: 0 g
- Sugar: 0 g
- Protein: 1 g

25. Parsley Root Veg Stew

Preparation time: 5 minutes
Cooking time: 35 - 40 minutes
Servings: 4

Ingredients:
- 2 garlic cloves
- 2 cups white rice
- 1 tsp. ground cumin
- 1 diced onion
- 2 cups water
- 4 peeled and diced turnips
- 1 tsp. cayenne pepper
- ¼ cup chopped fresh parsley
- ½ tsp. ground cinnamon
- 2 tbsps. olive oil
- 1 tsp. ground ginger
- 2 peeled and diced carrots

Direction:

1. In a large pot, heat the oil on a medium high heat before sautéing the onion for 4-5 minutes until soft.
2. Add the turnips and cook for 10 minutes or until golden brown.
3. Add the garlic, cumin, ginger, cinnamon, and cayenne pepper, cooking for a further 3 minutes.
4. Add the carrots and stock to the pot and then bring to the boil.
5. Turn the heat down to medium heat, cover and simmer for 20 minutes.
6. Meanwhile add the rice to a pot of water and bring to the boil.
7. Turn down to simmer for 15 minutes.
8. Drain and place the lid on for 5 minutes to steam.
9. Garnish the root vegetable stew with parsley to serve alongside the rice.

Nutrition:

- Calories: 210 kcal
- Total Fat: 7 g
- Saturated Fat: 0 g
- Cholesterol: 0 mg
- Sodium: 67 mg
- Total Carbs: 32 g
- Fiber: 0 g
- Sugar: 0 g
- Protein: 4 g

VEGETABLES

26.   Thai Tofu Broth

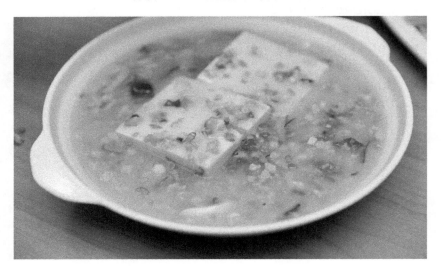

Preparation time: 5 minutes
Cooking time: 15 minutes
Servings: 4

Ingredients:

- 1 cup rice noodles
- ½ sliced onion
- 6 oz. drained, pressed and cubed tofu
- ¼ cup sliced scallions
- ½ cup water
- ½ cup canned water chestnuts
- ½ cup rice milk
- 1 tbsp. lime juice
- 1 tbsp. coconut oil
- ½ finely sliced chili
- 1 cup snow peas

Direction:

1. Heat the oil in a wok on a high heat and then sauté the tofu until brown on each side.
2. Add the onion and sauté for 2-3 minutes.
3. Add the rice milk and water to the wok until bubbling.
4. Lower to medium heat and add the noodles, chili and water chestnuts.
5. Allow to simmer for 10-15 minutes and then add the sugar snap peas for 5 minutes.
6. Serve with a sprinkle of scallions.

Nutrition:

- Calories: 304 kcal
- Total Fat: 13 g
- Saturated Fat: 0 g
- Cholesterol: 0 mg
- Sodium: 36 mg
- Total Carbs: 38 g
- Fiber: 0 g
- Sugar: 0 g
- Protein: 9 g

27. Delicious Vegetarian Lasagne

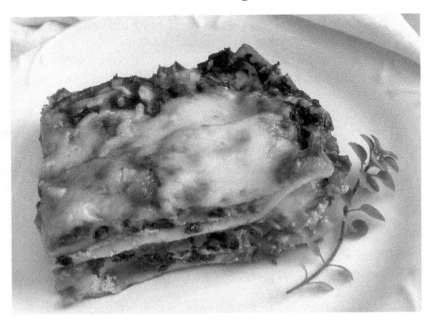

Preparation time: 10 minutes
Cooking time: 1 hour
Servings: 4

Ingredients:

- 1 tsp. basil
- 1 tbsp. olive oil
- ½ sliced red pepper
- 3 lasagna sheets
- ½ diced red onion
- ¼ tsp. black pepper
- 1 cup rice milk
- 1 minced garlic clove
- 1 cup sliced eggplant
- ½ sliced zucchini
- ½ pack soft tofu
- 1 tsp. oregano

Direction:

1. Preheat oven to 325 F/Gas Mark 3.
2. Slice zucchini, eggplant and pepper into vertical strips.
3. Add the rice milk and tofu to a food processor and blitz until smooth. Set aside.
4. Heat the oil in a skillet over medium heat and add the onions and garlic for 3-4 minutes or until soft.
5. Sprinkle in the herbs and pepper and allow to stir through for 5-6 minutes until hot.
6. Into a lasagne or suitable oven dish, layer 1 lasagna sheet, then 1/3 the eggplant, followed by 1/3 zucchini, then 1/3 pepper before pouring over 1/3 of tofu white sauce.
7. Repeat for the next 2 layers, finishing with the white sauce.
8. Add to the oven for 40-50 minutes or until veg is soft and can easily be sliced into servings.

Nutrition:

- Calories: 235 kcal
- Total Fat: 9 g
- Saturated Fat: 0 g
- Cholesterol: 0 mg
- Sodium: 35 mg
- Total Carbs: 10 g
- Fiber: 0 g
- Sugar: 0 g
- Protein: 5 g

28.   Chili Tofu Noodles

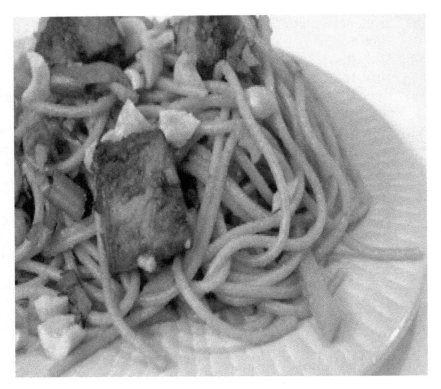

Preparation time: 5 minutes
Cooking Time: 15 minutes
Servings: 4

Ingredients:

- ½ diced red chili
- 2 cups rice noodles
- ½ juiced lime
- 6 oz. pressed and cubed silken firm tofu
- 1 tsp. grated fresh ginger
- 1 tbsp. coconut oil
- 1 cup green beans
- 1 minced garlic clove

Direction:

1. Steam the green beans for 10-12 minutes or according to package directions and drain.
2. Cook the noodles in a pot of boiling water for 10-15 minutes or according to package directions.
3. Meanwhile, heat a wok or skillet on a high heat and add coconut oil.
4. Now add the tofu, chili flakes, garlic and ginger and sauté for 5-10 minutes.
5. Drain the noodles and add to the wok along with the green beans and lime juice.
6. Toss to coat.
7. Serve hot!

Nutrition:

- Calories: 246 kcal
- Total Fat: 12 g
- Saturated Fat: 0 g
- Cholesterol: 0 mg
- Sodium: 25 mg
- Total Carbs: 28 g
- Fiber: 0 g
- Sugar: 0 g
- Protein: 10 g

29.   Curried Cauliflower

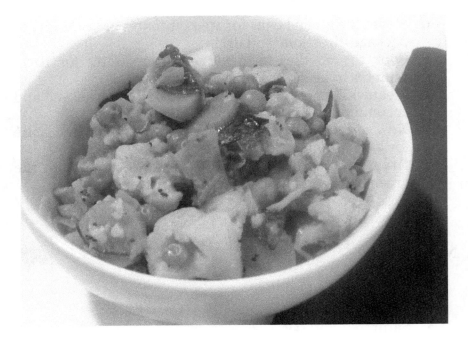

Preparation time: 5 minutes
Cooking time: 20 minutes
Servings: 4

Ingredients:

- 1 tsp. turmeric
- 1 diced onion
- 1 tbsp chopped fresh cilantro
- 1 tsp. cumin
- ½ diced chili
- ½ cup water
- 1 minced garlic clove
- 1 tbsp. coconut oil
- 1 tsp. garam masala
- 2 cups cauliflower florets

Direction:

1. Add the oil to a skillet on medium heat.
2. Sauté the onion and garlic for 5 minutes until soft.
3. Add the cumin, turmeric and garam masala and stir to release the aromas.
4. Now add the chili to the pan along with the cauliflower.
5. Stir to coat.
6. Pour in the water and reduce the heat to a simmer for
7. 15 minutes.
8. Garnish with cilantro to serve.

Nutrition:

- Calories: 108 kcal
- Total Fat: 7 g
- Saturated Fat: 0 g
- Cholesterol: 0 mg
- Sodium: 35 mg
- Total Carbs: 11 g
- Fiber: 0 g
- Sugar: 0 g
- Protein: 2 g

30.   Chinese Tempeh Stir Fry

Preparation time: 5 minutes
Cooking time: 15 minutes
Servings: 2

Ingredients:

- 2 oz. sliced tempeh
- 1 cup cooked brown rice
- 1 minced garlic clove
- ½ cup green onions
- 1 tsp. minced fresh ginger
- 1 tbsp. coconut oil
- ½ cup corn

Direction:

1. Heat the oil in a skillet or wok on a high heat and add the garlic and ginger.
2. Sauté for 1 minute.
3. Now add the tempeh and cook for 5-6 minutes before adding the corn for a further 10 minutes.
4. Now add the green onions and serve over brown rice.

Nutrition:

- Calories: 304 kcal
- Total Fat: 4 g
- Saturated Fat: 0 g
- Cholesterol: 0 mg
- Sodium: 91 mg
- Total Carbs: 35 g
- Fiber: 0 g
- Sugar: 0 g
- Protein: 10 g

FISH AND SEAFOOD

31.   Salmon & Pesto Salad

Preparation time: 5 minutes
Cooking time: 15 minutes
Servings: 2

Ingredients:

For the pesto:
- 1 minced garlic clove
- ½ cup fresh arugula
- ¼ cup extra virgin olive oi l
- ½ cup fresh basil
- 1 tsp. black pepper

For the salmon:
- 4 oz. skinless salmon fillet
- 1 tbsp. coconut oil
- For the salad:
- ½ juiced lemon
- 2 sliced radishes
- ½ cup iceberg lettuce
- 1 tsp. black pepper

Direction:

1. Prepare the pesto by blending all the ingredients for the pesto in a food processor or by grinding with a pestle and mortar. Set aside.
2. Add a skillet to the stove on medium-high heat and melt the coconut oil.
3. Add the salmon to the pan.
4. Cook for 7-8 minutes and turn over.
5. Cook for a further 3-4 minutes or until cooked through.

6. Remove fillets from the skillet and allow to rest.
7. Mix the lettuce and the radishes and squeeze over the juice of ½ lemon.
8. Flake the salmon with a fork and mix through the salad.
9. Toss to coat and sprinkle with a little black pepper to serve.

Nutrition:

Calories: 221 kcal
Total Fat: 34 g
Saturated Fat: 0 g
Cholesterol: 0 mg
Sodium: 80 mg
Total Carbs: 1 g
Fiber: 0 g
Sugar: 0 g
Protein: 13 g

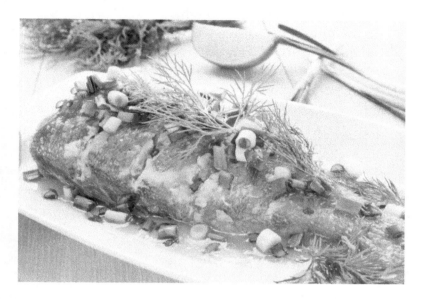

Preparation time: 5 minutes
Cooking time: 15 minutes
Servings: 2

Ingredients:

- 1 lemon
- ½ sliced fennel bulb
- 6 oz. sea bass fillets
- 1 tsp. black pepper
- 2 garlic cloves

Direction:

1. Preheat the oven to 375° F/Gas Mark 5.
2. Sprinkle black pepper over the Sea Bass.
3. Slice the fennel bulb and garlic cloves.
4. Add 1 salmon fillet and half the fennel and garlic to one sheet of baking paper or tin foil.
5. Squeeze in ½ lemon juices.

6. Repeat for the other fillet.
7. Fold and add to the oven for 12-15 minutes or until fish is thoroughly cooked through.
8. Meanwhile, add boiling water to your couscous, cover and allow to steam.
9. Serve with your choice of rice or salad.

Nutrition:

- Calories: 221 kcal
- Total Fat: 2 g
- Saturated Fat: 0 g
- Cholesterol: 0 mg
- Sodium: 119 mg
- Total Carbs: 3 g
- Fiber: 0 g
- Sugar: 0 g
- Protein: 14 g

33. Lemon, Garlic & Cilantro Tuna And Rice

Preparation time: 5 minutes
Cooking time: 0 minute
Servings: 2

Ingredients:

- ½ cup arugula
- 1 tbsp. extra virgin olive oil
- 1 cup cooked rice
- 1 tsp. black pepper
- ¼ finely diced red onion
- 1 juiced lemon
- 3 oz. canned tuna
- 2 tbsps. Chopped fresh cilantro

Direction:

1. Mix the olive oil, pepper, cilantro and red onion in a bowl.
2. Stir in the tuna, cover and leave in the fridge for as long as possible (if
3. you can) or serve immediately.
4. When ready to eat, serve up with the cooked rice and arugula!

Nutrition:

- Calories: 221 kcal
- Total Fat: 7 g
- Saturated Fat: 0 g
- Cholesterol: 0 mg
- Sodium: 143 mg
- Total Carbs: 26 g
- Fiber: 0 g
- Sugar: 0 g
- Protein: 11 g

34.   Sardine Fish Cakes

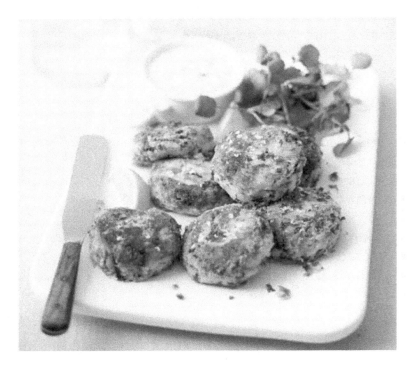

Preparation Time: 10 minutes
Cooking Time: 10 minutes
Servings: 4

Ingredients:

- 11 oz sardines, canned, drained
- 1/3 cup shallot, chopped
- 1 teaspoon chili flakes
- 1/2 teaspoon salt
- 2 tablespoon wheat flour, whole grain
- 1 egg, beaten
- 1 tablespoon chives, chopped
- 1 teaspoon olive oil
- 1 teaspoon butter

Directions:

1. Put the butter in the skillet and melt it.
2. Add shallot and cook it until translucent.
3. After this, transfer the shallot in the mixing bowl.
4. Add sardines, chili flakes, salt, flour, egg, chives, and mix up until smooth with the help of the fork.
5. Make the medium size cakes and place them in the skillet.
6. Add olive oil.
7. Roast the fish cakes for 3 minutes from each side over the medium heat.
8. Dry the cooked fish cakes with the paper towel if needed and transfer in the serving plates.

Nutrition:

- Calories: 221 kcal
- Total Fat: 12.2 g
- Saturated Fat: 0 g
- Cholesterol: 0 mg
- Sodium: 0 mg
- Total Carbs: 5.4 g
- Fiber: 0.1 g
- Sugar: 0 g
- Protein: 21.3 g

35. Cilantro And Lime Cod

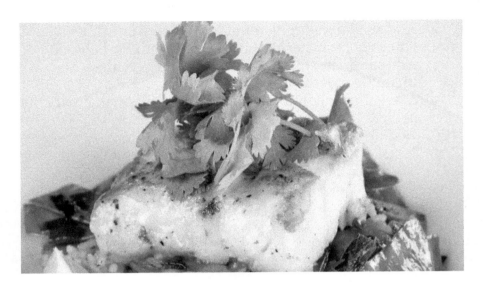

Preparation Time: 10 minutes
Cooking Time: 30 minutes
Servings: 4

Ingredients:

- 8 Tbsp. fresh cilantro
- .5 cup of mayonnaise
- 6 tsp. of lime juice
- 1 pound of cod fillets

Directions:

1. Combine the mayonnaise, lime juice, and cilantro. Transfer four Tbsp. of the combined ingredients to a smaller bowl to serve as sauce for the fish.
2. Brush the cod fillets with the remaining mixture.
3. Use canola oil spray and grease a frying pan. Fry the fillets over moderate temperature. Cook fish until firm but still moist. Serve with the remaining sauce.

Nutrition:

- Calories: 292 kcal
- Total Fat: 23 g
- Saturated Fat: 0 g
- Cholesterol: 57 mg
- Sodium: 228 mg
- Total Carbs: 1 g
- Fiber: 0 g
- Sugar: 0 g
- Protein: 20 g

MEAT AND POULTRY

36.   Baked Pork Chops

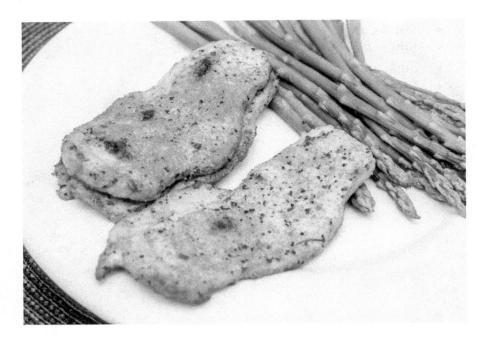

Preparation Time: 15 minutes
Cooking Time: 40 minutes
 Servings: 6

Ingredients:

- ½ cup flour
- 1 large egg
- ¼ cup water
- ¾ cup breadcrumbs
- 6 (3 ½ oz.) pork chops
- 2 tablespoons butter, unsalted
- 1 teaspoon paprika

Direction:

1. Begin by switching the oven to 350 degrees F to preheat.
2. Mix and spread the flour in a shallow plate.
3. Whisk the egg with water in another shallow bowl.
4. Spread the breadcrumbs on a separate plate.
5. Firstly, coat the pork with flour, then dip in the egg mix and then in the crumbs.
6. Grease a baking sheet and place the chops in it.
7. Drizzle the pepper on top and bake for 40 minutes.
8. Serve.

Nutrition:

- Calories: 221 kcal
- Total Fat: 7.8 g
- Saturated Fat: 1.9 g
- Cholesterol: 93 mg
- Sodium: 135 mg
- Total Carbs: 11.9 g
- Fiber: 3.5 g
- Sugar: 0.5 g
- Protein: 24.7 g

,

37.   Beef Kabobs With Pepper

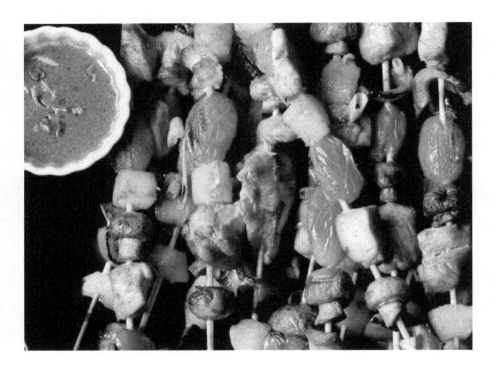

Preparation Time: 5 Minutes
 Cooking Time: 10 Minutes
Servings: 8

Ingredients:

- 1 Pound of beef sirloin
- ½ Cup of vinegar
- 2 tbsp of salad oil
- 1 Medium, chopped onion
- 2 tbsp of chopped fresh parsley
- ¼ tsp of black pepper
- 2 Cut into strips green peppers

Directions:

1. Trim the fat from the meat; then cut it into cubes of 1 and 1/2 inches each
2. Mix the vinegar, the oil, the onion, the parsley and the pepper in a bowl
3. Place the meat in the marinade and set it aside for about 2 hours; make sure to stir
4. from time to time.
5. Remove the meat from the marinade and alternate it on skewers instead with green pepper
6. Brush the pepper with the marinade and broil for about 10 minutes 4 inches from the heat
7. Serve and enjoy your kabobs

Nutrition:

- Calories: 357 kcal
- Total Fat: 24 g
- Saturated Fat: 0 g
- Cholesterol: 9 mg
- Sodium: 60 mg
- Total Carbs: 0 g
- Fiber: 2.3 g
- Sugar: 0 g
- Protein: 26 g

38.   One-Pot Beef Roast

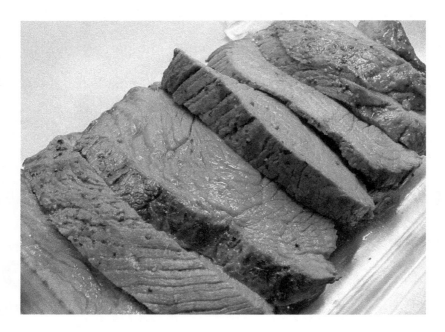

Preparation Time: 10 minutes
Cooking Time: 75 minutes
 Servings: 4

Ingredients:

- 3 ½ pounds beef roast
- 4 ounces mushrooms, sliced
- 12 ounces beef stock
- 1-ounce onion soup mix
- ½ cup Italian dressing

Direction:

1. Take a bowl and add the stock, onion soup mix, and Italian dressing
2. Stir
3. Put beef roast in pan

4. Add the mushrooms and stock mix to the pan and cover with foil
5. Preheat your oven to 300 °F
6. Bake for 1 hour and 15 minutes
7. Let the roast cool
8. Slice and serve
9. Enjoy the gravy on top!

Nutrition:

- Calories: 700 kcal
- Total Fat: 56 g
- Saturated Fat: 0 g
- Cholesterol: 0 mg
- Sodium: 0 mg
- Total Carbs: 10 g
- Fiber: 0 g
- Sugar: 0 g
- Protein: 70 g

,

39.   Cabbage And Beef Fry

Preparation Time: 5 minutes
 Cooking Time: 15 minutes
Servings: 4

Ingredients:

- 1 pound beef, ground
- ½ pound bacon
- 1 onion
- 1 garlic cloves, minced
- 1/2 head cabbage
- Salt and pepper to taste

Direction:

1. Take a skillet and place it over medium heat
2. Add chopped bacon, beef and onion until slightly browned
3. Transfer to a bowl and keep it covered
4. Add minced garlic and cabbage to the skillet and cook until slightly browned
5. Return the ground beef mixture to the skillet and simmer for 3-5 minutes over low heat
6. Serve and enjoy!

Nutrition:

- Calories: 360 kcal
- Total Fat: 22 g
- Saturated Fat: 0 g
- Cholesterol: 0 mg
- Sodium: 0 mg
- Total Carbs: 5 g
- Fiber: 0 g
- Sugar: 0 g
- Protein: 34 g

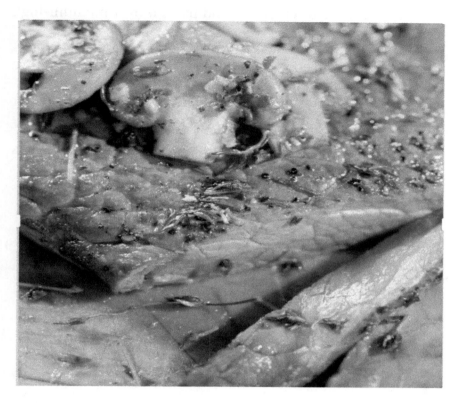

Preparation Time: 10 minutes
Cooking Time: 14 minutes
Servings: 4

Ingredients:

- 1 pound boneless beef sirloin steak, ¬æ inch thick, cut into 4 pieces
- 1 large red onion, chopped
- 1 cup mushrooms
- 4 garlic cloves, thinly sliced
- 4 tablespoons olive oil
- ½ cup green olives, coarsely chopped
- 1 cup parsley leaves, finely cut

Direction:

1. Take a large-sized skillet and place it over medium-high heat
2. Add oil and let it heat p
3. Add beef and cook until both sides are browned, remove beef and drain fat
4. Add the rest of the oil to skillet and heat it up
5. Add onions, garlic and cook for 2-3 minutes
6. Stir well
7. Add mushrooms olives and cook until mushrooms are thoroughly done
8. Return beef to skillet and lower heat to medium
9. Cook for 3-4 minutes (covered)
10. Stir in parsley
11. Serve and enjoy!

Nutrition:

- Calories: 386 kcal
- Total Fat: 30 g
- Saturated Fat: 0 g
- Cholesterol: 0 mg
- Sodium: 0 mg
- Total Carbs: 11 g
- Fiber: 0 g
- Sugar: 0 g
- Protein: 21 g

,

EGGS

41. Onion Cheese Omelet

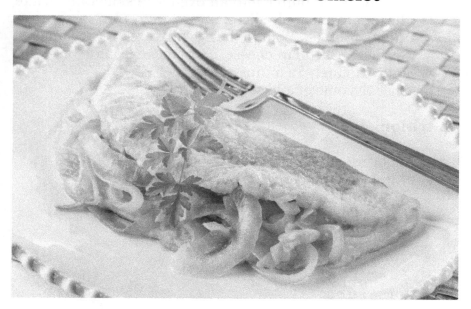

Preparation Time: 8 minutes
Cooking Time: 12 minutes
Servings: 2

Ingredients:

- 3 eggs
- ¼ cup liquid creamer
- 1 tablespoon water
- Black pepper to taste
- 1 tablespoon butter
- ¾ cup onion, sliced
- 1 large apple, peeled, cored, and sliced
- 2 tablespoons Cheddar cheese, grated

Direction:

1. Switch your gas oven to 400 degrees F to preheat.
2. Whisk the eggs with the liquid creamer, water, and black pepper in a suitable bowl.
3. Stir ¼ of the butter into an oven safe skillet and sauté the onion and apple slices.
4. After 5 minutes, pour in the egg mixture over the onions.
5. Sprinkle Cheddar cheese over the egg and bake for approximately 12 minutes.
6. Slice the omelet and serve.

Nutrition:

- Calories: 254 kcal
- Total Fat: 15.1 g
- Saturated Fat: 7.2 g
- Cholesterol: 268 mg
- Sodium: 184 mg
- Total Carbs: 20.7 g
- Fiber: 3.6 g
- Sugar: 1.4 g
- Protein: 10.9 g

42.   Mushroom Omelet

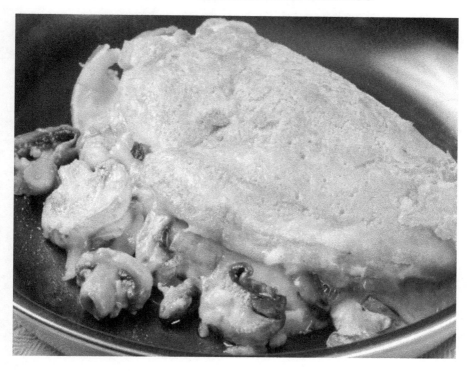

Preparation Time: 5 minutes
Cooking Time: 10 minutes
Servings: 2

Ingredients:

- 2 tablespoons and 1 teaspoon olive oil
- 1 shallot, minced
- ¼ lb. cremini mushrooms, rinsed
- Black pepper to taste
- 1 garlic clove, minced
- 2 teaspoons parsley, minced
- 4 eggs
- 1 tablespoon chives, minced
- 2 teaspoons milk
- 3 tablespoons Gruyere cheese, grated

Direction:

1. Set a suitable non-stick skillet over moderate heat and add 1 teaspoon olive oil.
2. Add in the shallot and mushrooms, then sauté for 5 minutes until soft.
3. Toss in the garlic and sauté for 1 minute.
4. Now add the rest of the oil to the same skillet.
5. Mix the eggs with the chives, milk, and black pepper in a bowl and pour it into the skillet.
6. Cook the egg omelet for about 2 minutes per side until golden brown then transfers to the serving place.
7. Serve with Gruyere cheese and parsley on top.
8. Enjoy.

Nutrition:

- Calories: 271 kcal
- Total Fat: 23 g
- Saturated Fat: 4.8 g
- Cholesterol: 328 mg
- Sodium: 208 mg
- Total Carbs: 4.8 g
- Fiber: 0.5 g
- Sugar: 2 g
- Protein: 13 g

43. Sausage & Egg Soup

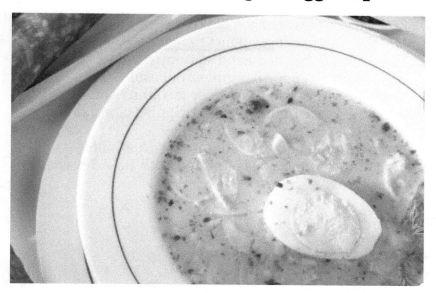

Preparation Time: 15 minutes
Cooking Time: 30 minutes
Servings: 4

Ingredients:

- ½ lb. ground beef
- Black pepper
- ½ teaspoon ground sage
- ½teaspoon garlic powder
- ½ teaspoon dried basil
- 4 slices bread (one day old), cubed
- 2 tablespoons olive oil
- 1 tablespoon herb seasoning blend
- 2 garlic cloves, minced
- 3 cups low-sodium chicken broth
- 1 cup water
- 4 tablespoons fresh parsley
- 4 eggs
- 2 tablespoons Parmesan cheese, grated

Direction:

1. Preheat your oven to 375 degrees F.
2. Mix the first five ingredients to make the sausage.
3. Toss bread cubes in oil and seasoning blend.
4. Bake in the oven for 8 minutes. Set aside.
5. Cook the sausage in a pan over medium heat.
6. Cook the garlic in the sausage drippings for 2 minutes.
7. Stir in the broth, water and parsley.
8. Bring to a boil and then simmer for 10 minutes.
9. Pour into serving bowls and top with baked bread, egg and sausage.

Nutrition:

- Calories: 335 kcal
- Total Fat: 19 g
- Saturated Fat: 0 g
- Cholesterol: 250 mg
- Sodium: 374 mg
- Total Carbs: 15 g
- Fiber: 0.9 g
- Sugar: 0 g
- Protein: 26 g

,

44.   Angel Eggs

Preparation Time: 30 minutes
Cooking Time: 0 minutes
 Servings: 2

Ingredients:

- 4 eggs, hardboiled and peeled
- 1 tablespoon vanilla bean sweetener, sugar-free
- 2 tablespoons Keto-Friendly mayonnaise
- 1/8 teaspoon cinnamon

Direction:

1. Halve the boiled eggs and scoop out the yolk
2. Place in a bowl
3. Add egg whites on a plate
4. Add sweetener, cinnamon, mayo to the egg yolks and mash
5. them well
6. Transfer the yolk mix to white halves
7. Serve and enjoy!

Nutrition:

- Calories: 184 kcal
- Total Fat: 15 g
- Saturated Fat: 0 g
- Cholesterol: 0 mg
- Sodium: 0 mg
- Total Carbs: 1 g
- Fiber: 0 g
- Sugar: 0 g
- Protein: 12 g

,

45.   Omelet

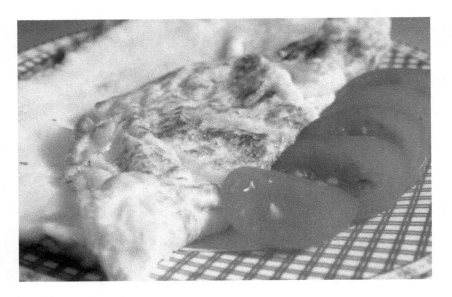

Preparation Time: 5 minutes
 Cooking Time: 5 minutes
Servings: 4

Ingredients

- 5 big of eggs
- 2 green onion, cleaved
- 1 tablespoon 2% of milk
- ¼ teaspoon dried basil
- ¼ teaspoon dried oregano
- Dash garlic powder
- Dash salt
- Dash pepper
- 2 tablespoon of butter
- ¼ cup disintegrated feta cheddar
- 2 cuts store ham, slashed
- 1 plum tomato, slashed
- 2 teaspoons balsamic vinaigrette

Directions:

1. In a little bowl, whisk eggs, green onion, milk, and seasonings until mixed. In an enormous nonstick skillet, heat margarine over medium-high warmth. Pour in egg blend. The blend should set promptly at the edge.
2. As eggs set, push cooked segments toward the middle, giving uncooked eggs a chance to stream underneath. At the point when eggs are thickened and no fluid egg stays, top one side with cheddar and ham.
3. Fold omelet down the middle; cut into two segments. Slide onto plates; top with tomato. Shower with vinaigrette before serving.

Nutrition:

- Calories: 289 kcal
- Total Fat: 20 g
- Saturated Fat: 0 g
- Cholesterol: 410 mg
- Sodium: 7490 mg
- Total Carbs: 0 g
- Fiber: 0 g
- Sugar: 0 g
- Protein: 21 g

,

DESSERTS

46.   Oatmeal And Berry Muffins

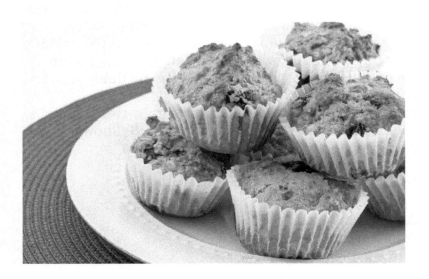

Preparation Time: 10 minutes
Cooking Time: 25 minutes
 Servings: 4

Ingredients:

- 1 cup (250 mL) non-blanched all-purpose flour
- 1/2 cup (125 mL) quick-cooking oatmeal 1/2 cup
- (160 mL) stuffed brown sugar
- 1/2 tbsp (1/2 cup) tea) baking soda
- 2 eggs
- 125 ml (1/2 cup) apple sauce
- 60 ml (1/4 cup)
- orange canola oil 1, grated rind only
- 1 lemon, grated rind
- 15 ml (1 tbsp) lemon juice
- 180 ml (3/4 cup) fresh raspberries (see note)
- 180 ml (3/4 cup) fresh blueberries (or blackberries)

———

Directions:

1. Put the grill at the center of the oven. Preheat oven to 180° C (350° F). Line
2. 12 muffin cups with paper or silicone trays.
3. In a bowl, combine flour, oatmeal, brown sugar, and baking soda. Book.
4. In a big bowl, whisk together eggs, applesauce, oil, citrus zest, and lemon juice. Add the dry ingredients to the wooden spoon. Add the berries and mix gently.
5. Spread the mixture in the boxes. Sprinkle top with pistachio muffins. Bake for 20 to 22 minutes or until a toothpick inserted in the center of a muffin comes out clean. Let cool.

Nutrition:

- Calories: 130.8 kcal
- Total Fat: 3 g
- Saturated Fat: 0.4 g
- Cholesterol: 31 mg
- Sodium: 93.8 mg
- Total Carbs: 24.1 g
- Fiber: 3.2 g
- Sugar: 10.1 g
- Protein: 3.7 g

47.   Crunchy Blueberry And Apples

Preparation Time: 20 minutes
 Cooking Time: 2 hours
Servings: 3

Ingredients:

- Crunchy
- 1 cup (1¼ cup) quick-cooking oatmeal
- ¼ cup (60 mL) brown sugar
- ¼ cup (60 mL) unbleached all-purpose flour
- 90 ml (6 tablespoons) melted margarine
- Garnish
- 125 ml (½ cup) brown sugar
- 20 ml (4 teaspoons) cornstarch
- 1 liter (4 cups) fresh or frozen blueberries (not thawed)
- 500 ml (2 cups) grated apples
- 1 Tbsp.
- (15 mL) melted margarine 15 mL (1 tablespoon) lemon juice

Directions:

1. Put the grill at the center of the oven. Preheat oven to 180 °C (350 °F)
2. In a bowl, mix dry ingredients. Add the margarine and mix until the mixture is just moistened. Book.
3. In a 20-cm (8-inch) square baking pan, combine brown sugar and cornstarch. Add the fruits, margarine, lemon juice, and mix well.
4. Cover with crisp and bake between 55 minutes and 1 hour, or until the crisp is golden brown.
5. Serve warm or cold.

Nutrition:

- Calories: 221 kcal
- Total Fat: 9.1 g
- Saturated Fat: 5.4 g
- Cholesterol: 21.6 mg
- Sodium: 160.6 mg
- Total Carbs: 34 g
- Fiber: 2.4 g
- Sugar: 9.5 g
- Protein: 2.5 g

48.   Raspberry Feast Meringue With Cream Diplomat

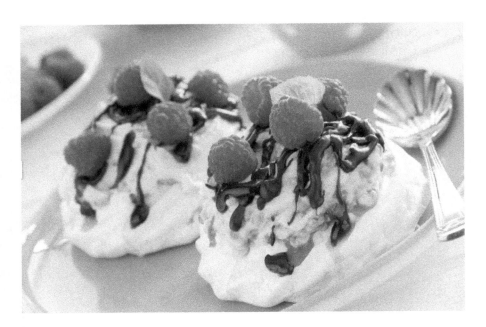

Preparation Time: 30 minutes
Cooking Time: 2 hours
 Servings: 4

Ingredients:

- Preparation of meringue
- 2 egg whites
- 1/2 cup caster sugar
- 1/4 tsp. vanilla extract
- 1/4 cup crumbled barley sugar
- Raspberry mousse preparation
- 1 cup frozen raspberries
- 1/4 cup water
- 2 tbsp. Raspberry Jell-O Powder with No Added Sugar
- 1 1/2 cup Cool Whip
- 1 bowl fresh raspberries

Directions:

1. To make the meringue, preheat the oven to 350 o F (175 o C) and line a baking sheet with parchment paper.
2. In a blender or bowl, whisk egg whites until the foam is obtained. Gently add the sugar while whisking until you get firm, shiny picks. Stir in vanilla extract and crumbled barley sugar.
3. Shape the meringues on the coated cookie sheet and place in the preheated oven. Turn off the oven and wait 2 hours. Do not open the oven. Once the meringues are dry, break the meringues into small bites.
4. To make the mousse, put frozen raspberries and water in a small saucepan. Heat until raspberries melt and are tender. Put these raspberries in a blender. Add the Jell-O powder and mix. Once the raspberries have completely cooled, incorporate the Cool Whip.
5. To shape the raspberry, place in balloon glasses for individual portions or in a large cake pan first a layer of raspberry mousse, then a layer of meringue, then fresh raspberries. Repeat the layers. Refrigerate for a few hours before serving.

Nutrition:

- Calories: 282.4 kcal
- Total Fat: 15.4 g
- Saturated Fat: 9.5 g
- Cholesterol: 56.3 mg
- Sodium: 18.1 mg
- Total Carbs: 34.6 g
- Fiber: 2.6 g
- Sugar: 29.2 g
- Protein: 3.2 g

49. Cheesecake Mousse With Raspberries

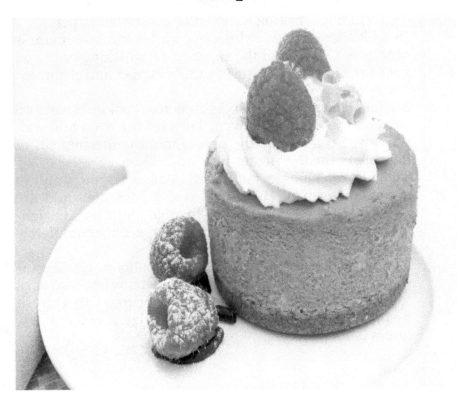

Preparation Time: 30 minutes
Cooking Time: 0 minutes
Servings: 6

Ingredients

- 1 cup light lemonade filling
- 1 can 8 oz cream cheese at room temperature
- ¾ cup SPLENDA no-calorie sweetener pellets
- 1 tbsp. at t. of lemon zest
- 1 tbsp. at t. vanilla extract
- 1 cup fresh or frozen raspberries

Direction:

1. Beat the cream cheese until it is sparkling; add ½ cup SPLENDA
2. Granules and mix until melted. Stir in lemon zest and vanilla.

3. Reserve some raspberries for decoration. Crush the rest of the raspberries with a fork and mix them with ¼ cup SPLENDA pellets until they are melted.
4. Lightly add the lump and cheese filling, and then gently but quickly add crushed raspberries. Share this mousse in 6 ramekins with a spoon and keep in the refrigerator until tasting.
5. Garnish mousses with reserved raspberries and garnish with fresh mint before serving.

Nutrition:

- Calories: 91.1 kcal
- Total Fat: 0.6 g
- Saturated Fat: 0.2 g
- Cholesterol: 2.5 mg
- Sodium: 95.6 mg
- Total Carbs: 15.9 g
- Fiber: 3.7 g
- Sugar: 8.8 g
- Protein: 7.4 g

50. Almond Meringue Cookies

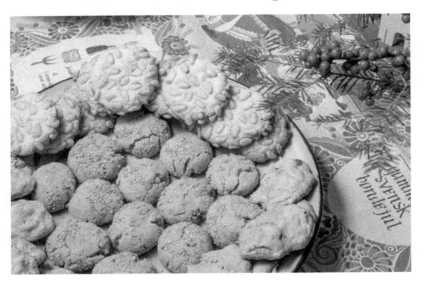

Preparation Time: 10 minutes
Cooking Time: 25 minutes
Servings: 4

Ingredients:

- 2 egg whites or 4 tbsp. pasteurized egg whites (at room temperature)
- 1 Tbsp. tartar cream

- ½ teaspoon almond extract vanilla extract
- ½ cup white sugar

Directions:

1. Preheat the oven to 300F.
2. Whisk the egg whites with the cream of tartar until the volume has doubled. Add other ingredients and whip until peaks form.
3. Using two teaspoons, drop a spoonful of meringue onto parchment paper with the back of the other spoon.
4. Bake at 300 F for about 25 minutes or until the meringues are crisp. Place in an airtight container.

Nutrition:

- Calories: 15 kcal
- Total Fat: 0 g
- Saturated Fat: 0 g
- Cholesterol: 0 mg
- Sodium: 3 mg
- Total Carbs: 3 g
- Fiber: 0 g
- Sugar: 2 g
- Protein: 0 g